This book belongs to:

phone

email

THIS BOOK PLANTS ONE TREE
ONE TREE PLANTED

THING OLOGY

The RN Pocket Notebook

ISBN: 978-1-959848-06-6
www.thing-ology.com

If you would like to help improv k
please reach out to us on www.t y.com

Where is your pain?

Où as-tu mal?

¿Dón de está tu dolor?

Wo hast du Schmerzen?

你的痛苦在哪里？

kde je tvoje bolest?

Hvor er din smerte?

Neren acıyor?

Var har du ont?

Де твій біль?

Dov'è il tuo dolore?

あなたの痛みはどこにありますか？

당신의 고통은 어디에 있습니까?

[1] [2] [3] [4] [5]

[6] [7] [8] [9] [10]

Do Not Use	Potential Problem	Use Instead
U, u (unit)	Mistaken for “0” (zero), the number “4” (four) or “cc”	Write “unit”
IU (International Unit)	Mistaken for IV (intravenous) or the number 10 (ten)	Write “International Unit”
Q.D., QD, q.d., qd (daily)	Mistaken for each other	Write “daily”
Q.O.D., QOD, q.o.d., qod (every other day)	Period after the Q mistaken for "I" and “O” mistaken for “I”	Write “every other day”
Trailing zero (X.0 mg)	Decimal point is missed	Write X mg
Lack of leading zero (.X mg)	Decimal point is missed	Write 0.X mg
MS	Can mean morphine sulfate or magnesium sulfate	Write “morphine sulfate” or write “magnesium sulfate”
MSO_4 and $MgSO_4$	Confused for one another	

2023

January

M	T	W	T	F	S	S
						1
2	3	4	5	6	7	8
9	10	11	12	13	14	15
16	17	18	19	20	21	22
23	24	25	26	27	28	29
30	31					

February

M	T	W	T	F	S	S
		1	2	3	4	5
6	7	8	9	10	11	12
13	14	15	16	17	18	19
20	21	22	23	24	25	26
27	28					

March

M	T	W	T	F	S	S
		1	2	3	4	5
6	7	8	9	10	11	12
13	14	15	16	17	18	19
20	21	22	23	24	25	26
27	28	29	30	31		

April

M	T	W	T	F	S	S
					1	2
3	4	5	6	7	8	9
10	11	12	13	14	15	16
17	18	19	20	21	22	23
24	25	26	27	28	29	30

May

M	T	W	T	F	S	S
1	2	3	4	5	6	7
8	9	10	11	12	13	14
15	16	17	18	19	20	21
22	23	24	25	26	27	28
29	30	31				

June

M	T	W	T	F	S	S
			1	2	3	4
5	6	7	8	9	10	11
12	13	14	15	16	17	18
19	20	21	22	23	24	25
26	27	28	29	30		

July

M	T	W	T	F	S	S
					1	2
3	**4**	5	6	7	8	9
10	11	12	13	14	15	16
17	18	19	20	21	22	23
24	25	26	27	28	29	30
31						

August

M	T	W	T	F	S	S
	1	2	3	4	5	6
7	8	9	10	11	12	13
14	15	16	17	18	19	20
21	22	23	24	25	26	27
28	29	30	31			

September

M	T	W	T	F	S	S
				1	2	3
4	5	6	7	8	9	10
11	12	13	14	15	16	17
18	19	20	21	22	23	24
25	26	27	28	29	30	

October

M	T	W	T	F	S	S
						1
2	3	4	5	6	7	8
9	10	11	12	13	14	15
16	17	18	19	20	21	22
23	24	25	26	27	28	29
30	31					

November

M	T	W	T	F	S	S
		1	2	3	4	5
6	7	8	9	**10**	11	12
13	14	15	16	17	18	19
20	21	22	**23**	24	25	26
27	28	29	30			

December

M	T	W	T	F	S	S
				1	2	3
4	5	6	7	8	9	10
11	12	13	14	15	16	17
18	19	20	21	22	23	24
25	26	27	28	29	30	31

Jan 1 • New Year's Day
Jan 2 • 'New Year's Day' day off
Jan 16 • Martin Luther King Jr. Day
Feb 14 • Valentine's Day
Feb 20 • Presidents' Day
Mar 17 • St. Patrick's Day
Apr 9 • Easter Sunday
Apr 10 • Easter Monday
Apr 18 • Tax Day

May 5 • Cinco de Mayo
May 14 • Mother's Day
May 29 • Memorial Day
Jun 14 • Flag Day
Jun 18 • Father's Day
Jun 19 • Juneteenth
Jul 4 • Independence Day
Sep 4 • Labor Day
Oct 9 • Columbus Day

Oct 31 • Halloween
Nov 7 • Election Day
Nov 10 • 'Veterans Day' day off
Nov 11 • Veterans Day
Nov 23 • Thanksgiving Day
Nov 24 • Black Friday
Dec 24 • Christmas Eve
Dec 25 • Christmas Day
Dec 31 • New Year's Eve

VACATION [Y] [N]

January 2023

	1ST SHIFT	2ND SHIFT	3RD SHIFT	OT/OTHER
1 Sun •				
2 Mon •				
3 Tue				
4 Wed				
5 Thu				
6 Fri				
7 Sat				
8 Sun				
9 Mon				
10 Tue				
11 Wed				
12 Thu				
13 Fri				
14 Sat				
15 Sun				
16 Mon •				
17 Tue				
18 Wed				
19 Thu				
20 Fri				
21 Sat				
22 Sun				
23 Mon				
24 Tue				
25 Wed				
26 Thu				
27 Fri				
28 Sat				
29 Sun				
30 Mon				
31 Tue				

• **Jan 1,** New Year's Day • **Jan 2,** 'New Year's Day' day off • **Jan 16,** Martin Luther King Jr. Day

• **Federal Holidays** • **Local Holidays** •• **Multiple Events**

VACATION [Y] [N]

February 2023

	1ST SHIFT	2ND SHIFT	3RD SHIFT	OT/OTHER
1 Wed				
2 Thu				
3 Fri				
4 Sat				
5 Sun				
6 Mon				
7 Tue				
8 Wed				
9 Thu				
10 Fri				
11 Sat				
12 Sun				
13 Mon				
14 Tue •				
15 Wed				
16 Thu				
17 Fri				
18 Sat				
19 Sun				
20 Mon •				
21 Tue				
22 Wed				
23 Thu				
24 Fri				
25 Sat				
26 Sun				
27 Mon				
28 Tue				

• **Feb 14,** Valentine's Day • **Feb 20,** Presidents' Day

• Federal Holidays **• Local Holidays** **•: Multiple Events**

VACATION [Y] [N]

March 2023

	1ST SHIFT	2ND SHIFT	3RD SHIFT	OT/OTHER
1 Wed				
2 Thu				
3 Fri				
4 Sat				
5 Sun				
6 Mon				
7 Tue				
8 Wed				
9 Thu				
10 Fri				
11 Sat				
12 Sun				
13 Mon				
14 Tue				
15 Wed				
16 Thu				
17 Fri •				
18 Sat				
19 Sun				
20 Mon				
21 Tue				
22 Wed				
23 Thu				
24 Fri				
25 Sat				
26 Sun				
27 Mon				
28 Tue				
29 Wed				
30 Thu				
31 Fri				

• **Mar 17,** St. Patrick's Day

• **Federal Holidays** • **Local Holidays** •• **Multiple Events**

VACATION [Y] [N]

April 2023

	1ST SHIFT	2ND SHIFT	3RD SHIFT	OT/OTHER
1 Sat				
2 Sun				
3 Mon				
4 Tue				
5 Wed				
6 Thu				
7 Fri				
8 Sat				
9 Sun •				
10 Mon •				
11 Tue				
12 Wed				
13 Thu				
14 Fri				
15 Sat				
16 Sun				
17 Mon				
18 Tue •				
19 Wed				
20 Thu				
21 Fri				
22 Sat				
23 Sun				
24 Mon				
25 Tue				
26 Wed				
27 Thu				
28 Fri				
29 Sat				
30 Sun				

• **Apr 9,** Easter Sunday • **Apr 10,** Easter Monday • **Apr 18,** Tax Day

• **Federal Holidays** • **Local Holidays** •• **Multiple Events**

VACATION [Y] [N]

May 2023

	1ST SHIFT	2ND SHIFT	3RD SHIFT	OT/OTHER
1 Mon				
2 Tue				
3 Wed				
4 Thu				
5 Fri •				
6 Sat				
7 Sun				
8 Mon				
9 Tue				
10 Wed				
11 Thu				
12 Fri				
13 Sat				
14 Sun •				
15 Mon				
16 Tue				
17 Wed				
18 Thu				
19 Fri				
20 Sat				
21 Sun				
22 Mon				
23 Tue				
24 Wed				
25 Thu				
26 Fri				
27 Sat				
28 Sun				
29 Mon •				
30 Tue				
31 Wed				

• **May 5,** Cinco de Mayo • **May 14,** Mother's Day • **May 29,** Memorial Day

• **Federal Holidays** • **Local Holidays** •• **Multiple Events**

VACATION [Y] [N]

June 2023

	1ST SHIFT	2ND SHIFT	3RD SHIFT	OT/OTHER
1 Thu				
2 Fri				
3 Sat				
4 Sun				
5 Mon				
6 Tue				
7 Wed				
8 Thu				
9 Fri				
10 Sat				
11 Sun				
12 Mon				
13 Tue				
14 Wed •				
15 Thu				
16 Fri				
17 Sat				
18 Sun •				
19 Mon •				
20 Tue				
21 Wed				
22 Thu				
23 Fri				
24 Sat				
25 Sun				
26 Mon				
27 Tue				
28 Wed				
29 Thu				
30 Fri				

• **Jun 14,** Flag Day • **Jun 18,** Father's Day • **Jun 19,** Juneteenth

• **Federal Holidays** • **Local Holidays** •• **Multiple Events**

VACATION [Y] [N]

July 2023

	1ST SHIFT	2ND SHIFT	3RD SHIFT	OT/OTHER
1 Sat				
2 Sun				
3 Mon				
4 Tue •				
5 Wed				
6 Thu				
7 Fri				
8 Sat				
9 Sun				
10 Mon				
11 Tue				
12 Wed				
13 Thu				
14 Fri				
15 Sat				
16 Sun				
17 Mon				
18 Tue				
19 Wed				
20 Thu				
21 Fri				
22 Sat				
23 Sun				
24 Mon				
25 Tue				
26 Wed				
27 Thu				
28 Fri				
29 Sat				
30 Sun				
31 Mon				

• **Jul 4,** Independence Day

• **Federal Holidays** • **Local Holidays** •• **Multiple Events**

VACATION [Y] [N]

August 2023

	1ST SHIFT	2ND SHIFT	3RD SHIFT	OT/OTHER
1 Tue				
2 Wed				
3 Thu				
4 Fri				
5 Sat				
6 Sun				
7 Mon				
8 Tue				
9 Wed				
10 Thu				
11 Fri				
12 Sat				
13 Sun				
14 Mon				
15 Tue				
16 Wed				
17 Thu				
18 Fri				
19 Sat				
20 Sun				
21 Mon				
22 Tue				
23 Wed				
24 Thu				
25 Fri				
26 Sat				
27 Sun				
28 Mon				
29 Tue				
30 Wed				
31 Thu				

VACATION [Y] [N]

September 2023

	1ST SHIFT	2ND SHIFT	3RD SHIFT	OT/OTHER
1 Fri				
2 Sat				
3 Sun				
4 Mon •				
5 Tue				
6 Wed				
7 Thu				
8 Fri				
9 Sat				
10 Sun				
11 Mon				
12 Tue				
13 Wed				
14 Thu				
15 Fri				
16 Sat				
17 Sun				
18 Mon				
19 Tue				
20 Wed				
21 Thu				
22 Fri				
23 Sat				
24 Sun				
25 Mon				
26 Tue				
27 Wed				
28 Thu				
29 Fri				
30 Sat				

• **Sep 4,** Labor Day

• **Federal Holidays** • **Local Holidays** •• **Multiple Events**

VACATION [Y] [N]

October 2023

	1ST SHIFT	2ND SHIFT	3RD SHIFT	OT/OTHER
1 Sun				
2 Mon				
3 Tue				
4 Wed				
5 Thu				
6 Fri				
7 Sat				
8 Sun				
9 Mon •				
10 Tue				
11 Wed				
12 Thu				
13 Fri				
14 Sat				
15 Sun				
16 Mon				
17 Tue				
18 Wed				
19 Thu				
20 Fri				
21 Sat				
22 Sun				
23 Mon				
24 Tue				
25 Wed				
26 Thu				
27 Fri				
28 Sat				
29 Sun				
30 Mon				
31 Tue •				

• **Oct 9,** Columbus Day • **Oct 31,** Halloween

• **Federal Holidays** • **Local Holidays** •• **Multiple Events**

VACATION [Y] [N]

November 2023

	1ST SHIFT	2ND SHIFT	3RD SHIFT	OT/OTHER
1 Wed				
2 Thu				
3 Fri				
4 Sat				
5 Sun				
6 Mon				
7 Tue •				
8 Wed				
9 Thu				
10 Fri •				
11 Sat •				
12 Sun				
13 Mon				
14 Tue				
15 Wed				
16 Thu				
17 Fri				
18 Sat				
19 Sun				
20 Mon				
21 Tue				
22 Wed				
23 Thu •				
24 Fri •				
25 Sat				
26 Sun				
27 Mon				
28 Tue				
29 Wed				
30 Thu				

• **Nov 7,** Election Day • **Nov 10,** 'Veterans Day' day off • **Nov 11,** Veterans Day • **Nov 23,** Thanksgiving Day • **Nov 24,** Black Friday

• **Federal Holidays** • **Local Holidays** •• **Multiple Events**

VACATION [Y] [N]

December 2023

	1ST SHIFT	2ND SHIFT	3RD SHIFT	OT/OTHER
1 Fri				
2 Sat				
3 Sun				
4 Mon				
5 Tue				
6 Wed				
7 Thu				
8 Fri				
9 Sat				
10 Sun				
11 Mon				
12 Tue				
13 Wed				
14 Thu				
15 Fri				
16 Sat				
17 Sun				
18 Mon				
19 Tue				
20 Wed				
21 Thu				
22 Fri				
23 Sat				
24 Sun •				
25 Mon •				
26 Tue				
27 Wed				
28 Thu				
29 Fri				
30 Sat				
31 Sun •				

• **Dec 24,** Christmas Eve • **Dec 25,** Christmas Day • **Dec 31,** New Year's Eve

• **Federal Holidays** • **Local Holidays** •• **Multiple Events**

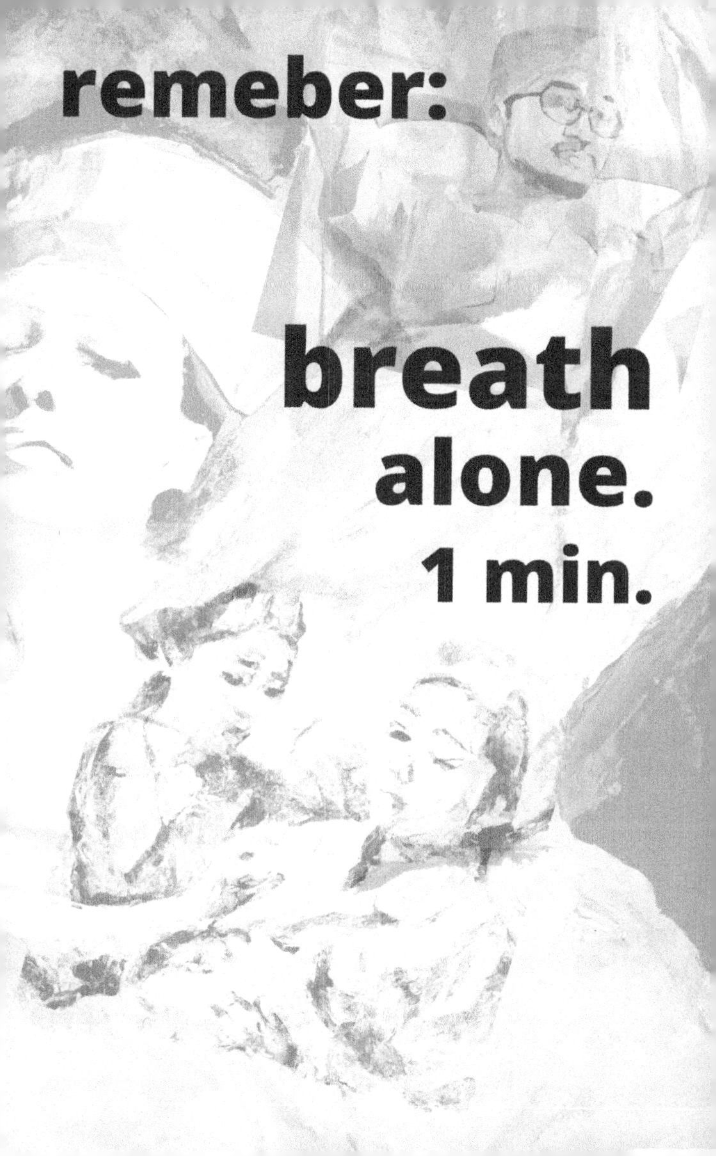
remeber:
breath
alone.
1 min.

rm# | time & date ___/___/___

task

☐

☐

☐

☐

☐

☐

☐

rm

___/___/___

☐

☐

☐

☐

☐

☐

☐

rm

___/___/___

☐

☐

☐

☐

☐

☐

☐

rm

___/___/___

rm

___/___/___

☐

☐

☐

☐

☐

☐

☐

rm

___/___/___

rm

___/___/___

☐

☐

☐

☐

☐

☐

☐

rm

___/___/___

rm

___/___/___

☐

☐

☐

☐

☐

☐

☐

rm

___/___/___

☐

☐

☐

☐

☐

☐

☐

rm

___/___/___

☐

☐

☐

☐

☐

☐

☐

rm

___/___/___

☐

☐

☐

☐

☐

☐

☐

rm

___/___/___

☐

☐

☐

☐

☐

☐

☐

rm

___/___/___

☐

☐

☐

☐

☐

☐

☐

rm

___/___/___

☐

☐

☐

☐

☐

☐

☐

rm

___/___/___

☐

☐

☐

☐

☐

☐

☐

rm

___/___/___

☐

☐

☐

☐

☐

☐

☐

rm

___/___/___

☐

☐

☐

☐

☐

☐

☐

rm

___/___/___

rm

___/___/___

☐

☐

☐

☐

☐

☐

☐

rm

___/___/___

- [ ]
- [ ]
- [ ]
- [ ]
- [ ]
- [ ]
- [ ]

rm

___/___/___

☐

☐

☐

☐

☐

☐

☐

rm

___/___/___

☐

☐

☐

☐

☐

☐

☐

rm

___/___/___

☐

☐

☐

☐

☐

☐

☐

rm

___/___/___

☐

☐

☐

☐

☐

☐

☐

rm

___/___/___

☐

☐

☐

☐

☐

☐

☐

rm

___/___/___

☐

☐

☐

☐

☐

☐

☐

rm

___/___/___

☐

☐

☐

☐

☐

☐

☐

rm

___/___/___

☐

☐

☐

☐

☐

☐

☐

rm

___/___/___

☐

☐

☐

☐

☐

☐

☐

rm

___/___/___

☐

☐

☐

☐

☐

☐

☐

rm

___/___/___

☐

☐

☐

☐

☐

☐

☐

rm

___/___/___

☐

☐

☐

☐

☐

☐

☐

rm

___/___/___

☐

☐

☐

☐

☐

☐

☐

rm

___/___/___

rm

___/___/___

☐

☐

☐

☐

☐

☐

☐

rm

___/___/___

☐

☐

☐

☐

☐

☐

☐

rm

___/___/___

- [ ]
- [ ]
- [ ]
- [ ]
- [ ]
- [ ]
- [ ]

rm

___/___/___

☐

☐

☐

☐

☐

☐

☐

rm

___/___/___

☐

☐

☐

☐

☐

☐

☐

rm

____/____/____

☐

☐

☐

☐

☐

☐

☐

rm

___/___/___

☐

☐

☐

☐

☐

☐

☐

rm

___/___/___

☐

☐

☐

☐

☐

☐

☐

rm

___/___/___

☐

☐

☐

☐

☐

☐

☐

rm

___/___/___

☐

☐

☐

☐

☐

☐

☐

rm

___/___/___

☐

☐

☐

☐

☐

☐

☐

rm

___/___/___

☐

☐

☐

☐

☐

☐

☐

rm

___/___/___

☐

☐

☐

☐

☐

☐

☐

rm

___/___/___

☐

☐

☐

☐

☐

☐

☐

rm

___/___/___

☐

☐

☐

☐

☐

☐

☐

rm

___/___/___

☐

☐

☐

☐

☐

☐

☐

rm

___/___/___

☐

☐

☐

☐

☐

☐

☐

rm

___/___/___

☐

☐

☐

☐

☐

☐

☐

rm

___/___/___

☐

☐

☐

☐

☐

☐

☐

rm

___/___/___

☐

☐

☐

☐

☐

☐

☐

rm

___/___/___

☐

☐

☐

☐

☐

☐

☐

rm

___/___/___

rm

___/___/___

rm

___/___/___

☐

☐

☐

☐

☐

☐

☐

rm

___/___/___

☐

☐

☐

☐

☐

☐

☐

rm

___/___/___

☐

☐

☐

☐

☐

☐

☐

rm

___/___/___

☐

☐

☐

☐

☐

☐

☐

rm

___/___/___

☐

☐

☐

☐

☐

☐

☐

rm

___/___/___

☐

☐

☐

☐

☐

☐

☐

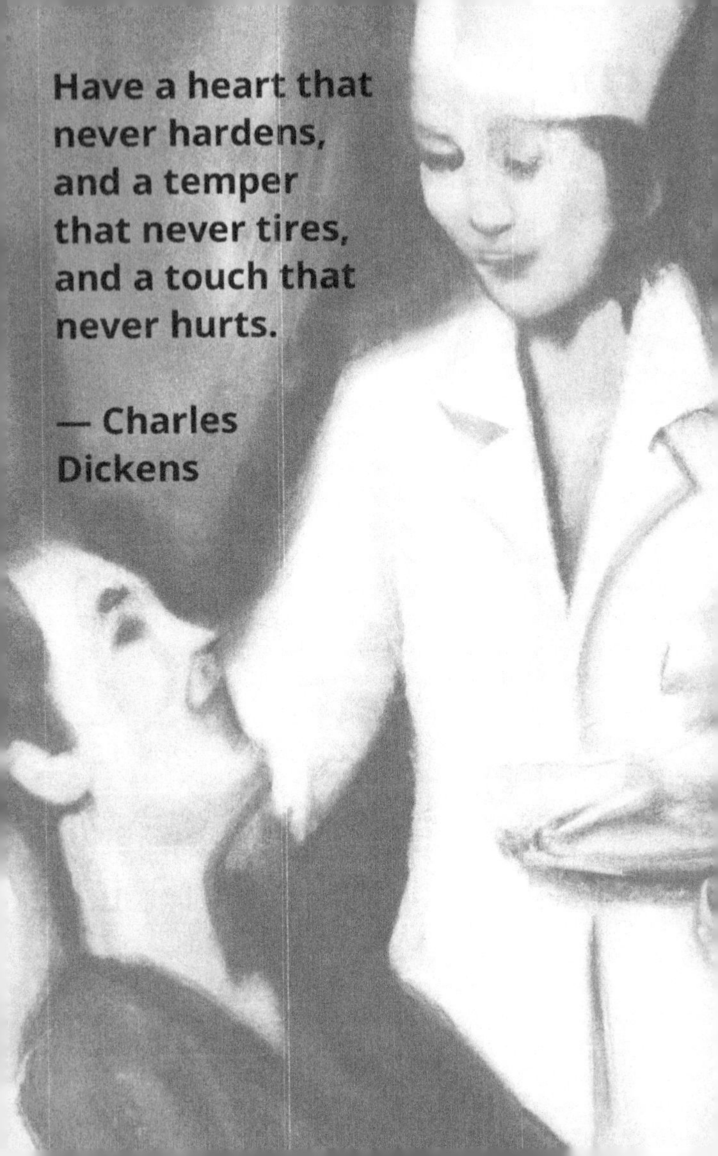
Have a heart that never hardens, and a temper that never tires, and a touch that never hurts.
— Charles Dickens

n:

rm____

time:

___ / ___

chief complaint

out of ordinary: **y__n__**

n: rm____

time: ____ / ____

chief complaint

out of ordinary: **y__n__**

n: rm____

time: ___ / ___

chief complaint

out of ordinary: **y**__**n**__

n: rm____

time: ____/____

chief complaint

out of ordinary: **y__n__**

n:

rm____

time:

____ / ____

chief complaint

out of ordinary: **y__n__**

n: rm____

time: ___ / ___

chief complaint

out of ordinary: **y**__**n**__

n:

rm____

time:

___ / ___

chief complaint

out of ordinary: **y__n__**

n: rm____

time: ___/___

chief complaint

out of ordinary: **y__n__**

n: rm____

time: ___ / ___

chief complaint

out of ordinary: **y**__**n**__

n: rm____

time: ____ / ____

chief complaint

out of ordinary: **y__n__**

n: rm____

time: ___ / ___

chief complaint

out of ordinary: **y__n__**

n: rm____

time: ___/___

chief complaint

out of ordinary: **y__n__**

n: rm____

time: ___ / ___

chief complaint

out of ordinary: **y__n__**

n: rm____

time: ___ / ___

chief complaint

out of ordinary: **y__n__**

n: rm____

time: ___ / ___

chief complaint

out of ordinary: **y__n__**

n: rm____

time: ___/___

chief complaint

out of ordinary: **y**__**n**__

n: rm____

time: ___ / ___

chief complaint

out of ordinary: **y**__ **n**__

n:

rm____

time:

____/____

chief complaint

out of ordinary: **y__n__**

n: rm____

time: ___ / ___

chief complaint

out of ordinary: **y__n__**

n: rm____

time: ____/____

chief complaint

out of ordinary: **y__n__**

n: rm____

time: ____/____

chief complaint

out of ordinary: **y__n__**

n: rm____

time: ____/____

chief complaint

out of ordinary: **y__n__**

n: rm____

time: ____ / ____

chief complaint

out of ordinary: **y**__ **n**__

n:

rm____

time:

___/___

chief complaint

out of ordinary: **y__n__**

n: rm____

time: ___ / ___

chief complaint

out of ordinary: **y__n__**

n: rm____

time: ____ / ____

chief complaint

out of ordinary: **y__n__**

n: rm____

time: ____ / ____

chief complaint

out of ordinary: **y**__**n**__

n:

rm____

time:

____/____

chief complaint

out of ordinary: **y__n__**

n:

rm____

time:

____ / ____

chief complaint

out of ordinary: **y**__**n**__

n: rm____

time: ___/___

chief complaint

out of ordinary: **y__n__**

n:

rm___

time:

___ / ___

chief complaint

out of ordinary: **y**__**n**__

n:

rm____

time:

___/___

chief complaint

out of ordinary: **y__n__**

n: rm____

time: ____ / ____

chief complaint

out of ordinary: **y**__**n**__

n: rm____

time: ____/____

chief complaint

out of ordinary: **y__n__**

n: rm____

time: ___ / ___

chief complaint

out of ordinary: **y__n__**

n: rm____

time: ___/___

chief complaint

out of ordinary: **y**__**n**__

n: rm____

time: ___ / ___

chief complaint

out of ordinary: **y__n__**

n: rm____

time: ___ / ___

chief complaint

out of ordinary: **y**__**n**__

notes

a

notes

a

notes

b

notes

b

notes

C

notes

C

notes

d

notes

d

notes

e

notes

e

notes

f

notes

notes

g

notes

g

notes

h

notes

h

notes

i

notes

i

notes

j

notes

j

notes

k

notes

notes

notes

notes

m

notes

m

notes

n

notes

n

notes

0

notes

0

notes

p

notes

p

notes

q

notes

q

notes

r

notes

r

notes

S

notes

S

notes

notes

t

notes

notes

u

notes

V

notes

V

notes

W

notes

W

notes

X

notes

X

notes

y

notes

y

notes

Z

notes

Z

Made in the USA
Monee, IL
08 November 2026

67379966R00132